How to Become
a Pharmacist

The Ultimate Guide
to a Successful Career
as a Pharmacist

by Gracie Elingston

Table of Contents

Introduction

Since its inception in the 19th century, the pharmaceutical industry was, and still is, one of the most flourishing and fastest growing industries in the world for the simple reason that people get sick. More diseases are being discovered every year, generating a constant need for new drugs. New drugs require great amounts of research and development, funded by the government, the private sector, or the pharmaceutical companies themselves. Research can take months, years, or even decades, and even then the drug must be approved by authorities such as the Food and Drug Administration (FDA). There are also trials which need to be done before submission to the authorities. Working in this industry can be painful, but it is very rewarding.

Historically, the pharmacist's main role was to check and distribute drugs to doctors. Their role has changed somewhat in modern times, and pharmacists are now also responsible for advising patients and health care providers on the drugs that they take. They are the middle man between the doctor who prescribes the drugs, and the patient. They also make sure that patients are coping well with the drugs they are prescribed. The modern pharmacist can even prescribe drugs themselves. They have to know all the different drugs, and understand the prescriptions written up by a doctor. This is a lot to learn, so why would anyone want to enter this profession?

First, people who graduate with a Pharmacy degree are some of the best-paid. Take for instance hospital staff pharmacists. These people earn up to $113,600 a year. Clinical and retail pharmacists earn about the same. The median salary and wage for all pharmacists in the US in May 2008 was $106,410, with the lowest 10 percent earning about $77,390, and the highest earning $131,440. Most employers will also give pharmacists health and retirement benefits.

Of course that level of salary can only be reached after intense training. Pharmacists have to understand biochemistry and the biochemical processes that happen when drugs are taken into the body. They have to appreciate and understand drugs as a whole, including their side effects, their intended uses and other properties they may have. Pharmacists will have to understand the human body, and what goes on there. This type of training cannot be covered in four years, and will require a doctorate degree. Pharmacists are able to practice without a doctorate degree in some countries, but their responsibilities are likely to be less than those of pharmacists in the United States.

Being a pharmacist can be very rewarding, both financially and in the ability to help others. In the following chapters, we'll discuss what it really takes to enter this prestigious field.

Chapter 1: Important Course Work and Preparation

If you want to realize your dream of becoming a pharmacist, first you will have to obtain a Bachelors Degree. Of course, in order to obtain a Bachelors Degree, you have to enter University. To do that, you will have to get your high school diploma, or you can bypass that and get a General Education Development (GED) certification.

Schools that offer pre-pharmacology programs tend to look for students with good or satisfactory GPAs, but they look particularly at how well you do in science courses. If you want to be a pharmacist, you cannot sleep through that Biology class! It pays to take more interest in what your teacher is saying, especially when it comes to anatomy and physiology. You will have to know how the body functions, as well as the different illnesses that spoil those functions. Pay close attention to where the different organs are in the body, and what each organ, tissue and cell does. You won't remember what every single tissue or even organ does in the body, but it pays to read up on them.

Biology is not the only subject you should pay attention to in class: Chemistry is another important discipline that is needed to enter a pre-pharmacology program in University. It may be that you struggle with one subject more than another, but it is important to pay equal attention to Chemistry. The human body is made up of thousands of different chemicals. When in University, you will have to learn Biochemistry, the chemistry of biological processes, but high school doesn't go into depth. With chemistry, you can learn about which processes produce heat, and which ones absorb it. You can understand the properties of water. You will understand the elements on the periodic table, and their properties. Why are these important to know and understand in pharmacology? Well, there are certain chemical reactions that happen in the body that cause fever, and some chemicals in drugs that can reduce temperature. Water makes up about 75% of the human body, so of course you will have to know the properties of water. Why the elements on the periodic table? Well, if you look at the nutritional contents on any pill bottle, you will see chemicals containing the names of elements such as lithium, carbon and calcium. All these elements have different properties that a pharmacist will need to know in order to understand how well they can come together to form the drug that is needed.

There are other subjects that you need to pay attention to, such as physics and mathematics. You won't have to know these subjects back to front, you're not expected to be Albert Einstein, but they are good supplementary subjects.

Pre-pharmacology colleges provide degrees in Biology, Biochemistry, and others, and they usually have the lowest acceptance rates out of all the colleges and faculties in the University. Admission departments will look at your school life, so you will need to stand out among your peers. Ensure that you are involved in school life, as they want to see how well you can handle the rounded life of a University student, especially as a science student. Ensure your grades are up. This is probably the most important thing, as they follow you right through life. However, if you graduated with a less-than-stellar GPA, you don't need to worry, as there are some colleges that will accept average GPAs. You can also use other options such as the GED if your GPA falls below average.

The General Education Development (GED) examination is comprised of four or five subjects in which the student is tested in science, mathematics, social studies, reading and writing. You can take this test if you are not comfortable going back to high school to achieve your diploma, or if your GPA was not very good. You will be asked questions that an average student would be expected to know in the American public school system, hence it pays to know as much as possible. But what if you don't know, and you don't want to go back to a high school class? Well, there are many institutions and businesses, both small and large, which are happy to support those who want to do classes at the times that they feel fit. You can simply search for the institutions that offer GED prep classes on the internet, and visit their offices.

There's also the matter of your SATs and/or ACTs. These examinations are needed to enter college. The SAT is the most common college placement examination in the country. The three subjects administered in these tests are Reading, Math and Writing. Each subject is graded on a scale of 200-800. Minimum acceptance scores vary between colleges and college departments, and can range from 400 to over 700. If you have a weak GPA but stellar SAT scores, pre-pharmacology colleges are more likely to accept you. It is harder to tell if it's the other way around, although your GPA does carry a lot of weight when it comes to acceptance. Your SATs are all about your preparedness for University, while your GPA shows how well you did in high school. At the same time, you can't go through 4 years of high school and get high grades throughout without hard work. Preparations for SATs can be stressful. Some take extra classes on top of the ones they are already receiving at school to ensure they are fully prepared for their SATs. It must be noted however that a good GPA and satisfactory SATs will definitely get you into a good college or university.

Whatever steps you decide to take, ensure that you are well-equipped, as these tests can be cruelly punishing to those who are not properly prepared. Take as many classes as you need, especially in areas in which you feel you are weakest. A good pharmacologist will need to be strong in all the areas tested in the GED and SAT. Make sure that the science area is the strongest in your GED, that math is the strongest in your SATs. Reading and writing are mainly about aptitude, and will take practice more than studying to perfect.

Chapter 2: Graduate with First Degree

Now that you have your diploma and/or GED, and have satisfactory scores in your SATs, it's time to enter college to get that degree! Always make sure to choose a program that has pre-pharmacy coursework in it. Yes coursework. The good news is that you don't have to complete a straight science degree if you don't want to. You will have to achieve good high school science grades to ensure that you can take courses offered by science departments in college, but the fact is you can choose any four-year program your heart desires. The amount of science coursework needed to enter a pharmacology program is two years worth of core science courses. Therefore, if you want to do a degree in Law, you must take science coursework along with it for the first two years. It's better to do it in the first two years, because you have less stressful work to do in your Freshman and Sophomore years, plus you may only be allowed to do major coursework in science for the first two years of that program. The courses must revolve around human anatomy and physiology, biology, chemistry, physics, psychology and calculus.

There are some schools that offer a tailor-made pre-pharmacy program. You will obtain a Bachelor of Science in Pre-pharmacy. Not all Universities provide these programs however, and you will have to find a University near you that does. Call a University near you and ask them what the options are, or look on their website. The operator will forward you to the science department, where you can ask them what the best options are for you to enter Pharmacology. The best degrees are typically Biology, Biochemistry, and Chemistry. These degrees can be used anywhere and, if you later decide to go to medical school instead of pharmacy school, you will still be able to with those degrees.

Many people go to University thinking that it will be a walk in the park. Even if you were smart in high school and breezed right through, there is a very high chance that University will not be the same. Getting through a tertiary-level of education takes immense commitment and, especially for a competitive degree in pharmacy, you will need to do a lot of studying to stay ahead of the curve. First year courses are mainly general, so you will mostly do courses like General Biology and General Chemistry. These courses cover every single facet you will study throughout your tenure at University, but in a more simplified manner. These courses are usually the ones that are set to weed out the "tares", especially during the second semester. Again, to get through these courses, it all depends on your level of commitment to the program.

As was said before, you don't have to do a straight science degree, but you do need two years worth of science coursework in your transcript. Depending on your major course of study, you may find that the science coursework is best done at the beginning. In other degrees it may be best to wait until the end. However the two years of coursework will almost always be from the first two years of a program offered by that college/department. Talk to your college advisor and they will guide you in the way you should go.

When you have reached your third year, it will be time to start thinking about your post-graduate studies. You will have to start preparing for your PCATs, which are the tests you will take in order for you to enter the pharmacy program of your choice. There are some schools that don't require PCATs, but these are in the minority. If you want to enter grad school immediately after you graduate, taking the PCATs in your third year is a must.

Applying is also important at this point in your college tenure. Choosing the right school to go to is hard, and will take into account many factors including location, rate of admission, social life, services and school prestige. There are approximately 130 pharmacy schools to choose from. If you're having a hard time choosing the right school, there is a service called the Pharmacy College Application

Service (PharmCAS) which allows you to apply to multiple schools. Not all schools use this program, however, so you will need to do your research. The application process begins right after you have received your PCAT scores, since you can't apply to PharmCAS without them.

Do not forget to have a life. As a matter of fact, graduate schools get applications with high GPAs and test scores all the time. What they want is someone who can contribute to their school in more ways than one. They want well-rounded people, not bookworms. Hence, make sure you play basketball. Or join the volleyball team. Or the debate club. Join the choir. Participate in some community outreach. All these things will show that you are a well-rounded individual.

So, we've already gone through 7-8 years of what it takes to become a pharmacist. Now it's time for the final 4 years.

Chapter 3: The PCAT

The Pharmacy College Admission Test, or PCAT, is a standardized test for students entering pharmacy school. Like many other admission tests, the PCAT tests out your verbal ability, quantitative ability, as well as your knowledge in chemistry and biology. You will also be tested for your reading comprehension and your writing.

This test is comprised of 232 multiple-choice questions, as well as several writing topics to choose from. As you can see, it is a very difficult test to do. However, if you want to pass this test with flying colors, there are some things that you can do to optimize your chances.

First of all, have the belief in yourself that you can do what is required of you. Believing in your life goals will give you the extra drive and motivation to complete what you started. Many people stop their courses simply because they do not believe in what they are doing. In order to get through these tests with a sane and sound mind, all worrying and doubt should be put behind you. Then you can move on to the next step.

As was said before, if you want to enter into pharmacy school immediately after you finish college, then your junior year is definitely the best time to do it. If not your junior year, then right at the beginning of your senior year. Many of these schools require applications a year before the opening semester, while some have deadlines the preceding semester. It all depends on the school and how many applications they will have to sift through. The more prestigious the school, the earlier the deadline is likely to be. Ensure that your PCAT studies do not interfere too much with your studies for school, as your GPA will still need to stay up. This is why many people choose to have a year or two off before they enter pharmacy school, so that they don't have to start preparations so early. It all depends on you and what you think you can handle.

Study regularly! Don't fall into the bad college habit of procrastination and cramming at the last minute. Cramming when you know time is short causes adrenaline to flow, your heart to race, and your mind to go into overdrive. The bad news is that the mind goes into overdrive spewing information out, rather than taking it in. This is why your mind is so foggy during study time, and when it's time to recollect the information. Also, practice. You can't study subjects like reading and comprehension. Those require that you know how to do them well, which will only come with practice. You will never be a master at understanding poems, novels and other literature if you never read a book. You will never become a master at writing short stories just by reading about it on the internet. It all takes practice.

While preparing, make sure that you have a proper studying space. This must be free of noise and distraction. Many people study with music, but the genre chosen must be conducive to study. Some people are able to study well with pop music blasting in their ears but, for most people, music with heavy beats cause a distraction. Classical music played at a low volume provides a perfect backdrop for studying.

Another good practice is to create new techniques for revision. It's not all about flash cards and blurting out an answer. There are many ways in which you can revise a chapter that you've been studying. If you find that you are not remembering much, you will have to go and study it again. So don't wait until you've gone through the whole book to start revising. Make sure you revise immediately after every chapter to make sure the information sticks.

Chapter 4: Graduate with a Pharmacology Degree

You've done well in your PCATs, and you have been accepted into your pharmacy school of choice. Congratulations! But it will only get harder from here. Completing a graduate program will require the same type of effort that the undergraduate program took. You will have to commit to your program of study and make sure that you know your material well, or else you will flunk out. Had you been studying in the United States before 2003, you would not have needed a Doctor of Pharmacy degree, but many developed countries are following suit in making the doctoral degree mandatory. This is because the pharmacist's role is growing as more diseases pop up. With more diseases come more drugs, and this makes it necessary for pharmacists to know a great deal. Advances in science and technology also require that the pharmacist is well versed in the business.

The Doctor of Pharmacy degree lasts about four years, give or take, depending on how you entered the school. Some enter the program through a six year accelerated program straight from high school, while most admit after two to three years of undergraduate studies. The Bachelor of Science in Pharmacy was the de facto degree for pharmacists in the country, but that was soon changed by regulating bodies. The BSc.

in Pharmacy is still the top degree in many countries around the world.

There are many schools in the country that offer degrees in pharmacy, approximately 130, in fact. There are many schools that offer an accelerated program, which include Appalachian College of Pharmacy, Ferris State University College of Pharmacy, Massachusetts College of Pharmacy and Health Sciences, Pacific University of Pharmacy, St. Joseph College of Pharmacy, among others. A simple Google search will give you what you're looking for.

There are some Universities that are accredited by the Accreditation Council for Pharmacy Education that offer part-time and online programs. These programs are however available only to those with a BSc in Pharmacy and a license to practice. If you did not take that route in college, this is not for you.

When you have been admitted, you can choose either to do the Pharm.D. program, or the PhD program. The PhD is all about research, and you will not be able to practice pharmacy with this degree. Some schools do not offer the PhD or M.Sc. programs, however, and will only offer the Pharm.D. programs. The Pharm.D. program goes into more depth than the B.Sc. Pharm.D. candidates must perform more hands-on clinical preparation, a year of clinical rotation in different healthcare settings, and greater emphasis on clinical pharmacy.

Once the program is done, it is time to graduate! What after graduation? Well, some graduates opt to do one to two years of residency. These residency programs are great as they give years of clinical experience in a short timeframe. This route is seen as a better way to enter the working world, as employers seem to favor those who have done residencies. Another route is for graduates to move on to do fellowships geared toward research. These fellowships can last anywhere from one to three years, requiring a year of residency.

Chapter 5: Get Licensed and Start Working

You have finished the long and arduous task of completing your studies, and now you want to get licensure to practice your trade. All pharmacists must have a license to practice. To receive a license, you will need to take the North American Pharmacist Licensure Examination, or NAPLEX for short, and also the Multi-state Pharmacy Jurisprudence Exam, or the MPJE.

The NAPLEX is a test that is administered by the National Association of Boards of Pharmacy (NABP). These tests make it easier for state boards to assess a pharmacist's aptitude and knowledge. It is an exclusively computer-administered exam, hence people can apply for an exam at any time and be able to do it two business days later. Each exam taker has about four hours to do the 185 questions. Only 150 of these 185 are marked. They do this to find which questions should be included or excluded from future tests. There is no way of telling which of these questions will be the ones omitted from marking.

The format consists of multiple choice questions, with no essays. The test is linear and there is no way of backtracking on an answer. Future questions will change depending on how you answer previous questions, in order to properly gauge your skill levels in different categories. You will be able to check your score seven days later, and you will need at least a 75 to pass. If you did not get above a 75, you will have 91 days until you can retake the test. There will also be a profile explaining the areas you fell short in and what needs more work.

The MBJE is only required for those living in Arkansas, California, Virginia, and four other states. It is best to check your state board to see which tests are needed in order for you to practice. When you receive your license, you will have to visit some government agencies in order for you to be assigned the title "Pharmacist" or "Registered Pharmacist."

The tests are complete! Now time to find a job. The most common workplaces for pharmacists include hospitals, grocery stores, drug stores, public health care agencies, schools and government agencies. It all depends on where you feel most comfortable. You may even choose to try out several different Pharmacy positions during the first few years of your career in order to help you discover what position is most suited to your tastes and career goals.

Conclusion

The road to a career in pharmacology is long, tiring and stressful but, in the end, it is worth it. You will be well-compensated and you will work in an industry that will continue to thrive as long as people keep getting sick – which they always will. Right now, and for the foreseeable future, working in pharmacy will give you the satisfaction of helping people recover from their condition. Let's summarize some of the points made.

Pharmacy is the science of making and distributing drugs. The pharmaceutical industry is one of the biggest industries in the world, worth hundreds of billions of dollars. Pharmacists are responsible for the administering of drugs to the patient, and also performing trials and observations where the drugs are concerned.

Pharmacy takes about 8 to 12 years from high school to becoming a practicing pharmacist. After receiving the Pharm.D. degree, the pharmacy candidate must take a number of tests in order for them to get a license to practice. Successful completion will make the candidate eligible to receive the title of "Pharmacist".

With a median salary of about $100,000, and added benefits including health and 401k, no wonder this field is looking more and more attractive to incumbents. The world needs pharmacists more than ever to combat evolving diseases.

Finally, I'd like to thank you for purchasing this book! If you enjoyed it or found it helpful, I'd greatly appreciate it if you'd take a moment to leave a review on Amazon. Thanks, and good luck with your Pharmacy career!

Made in the USA
San Bernardino, CA
21 August 2018